# Power Through Pain

# Power Through Pain

✦

## Living with Reflex Neurovascular Dystrophy

*1 injury*
*20 doctors*
*41 months*
*1200 days*

*Elizabeth Elster*

iUniverse, Inc.
New York  Lincoln  Shanghai

# Power Through Pain
## Living with Reflex Neurovascular Dystrophy

iUniverse books may be ordered through booksellers or by contacting:

iUniverse
2021 Pine Lake Road, Suite 100
Lincoln, NE 68512
www.iuniverse.com
1-800-Authors (1-800-288-4677)

Because of the dynamic nature of the Internet, any Web addresses or links contained in this book may have changed since publication and may no longer be valid.

The views expressed in this work are solely those of the author and do not necessarily reflect the views of the publisher, and the publisher hereby disclaims any responsibility for them.

Profits from this book will be donated to RND awareness, education, and research.

ISBN: 978-0-595-43716-0 (pbk)
ISBN: 978-0-595-88047-8 (ebk)

Printed in the United States of America

# Contents

# A Message to Those Who Suffer

**YOU ARE NOT ALONE.**

Do not turn one more page in this book thinking you are suffering by yourself. We are here, connected to you by an invisible web of compassion and strength. As fellow pain sufferers, we understand that living in chronic pain can be depressing, saddening, and infuriating. Please seek professional help if you are depressed. Find a local chronic pain support group or participate in internet chats and boards online where you can meet others in pain and receive their support.

*To all of you who suffer in pain every day:*
*Stay strong and never give up hope!*
*You are not alone.*

I saw Pain clearly.

She was angry and restless.

She turned and slowly menaced at me.

I saw her pale skin and tired eyes,

And heard her sit in the shadows and bellow.

And I felt her aching too.


By Martha Elster

# *Acknowledgments*

Thank you to my parents, especially my mom, for giving me strength and teaching me how to reach out to others. Thank you for always being there for me and never giving up until we found an answer.

Thank you to my sisters, Martha and Patricia, for showing me that I have a strong network of people who believe in me and who will always care for me no matter how much I may suffer.

Thank you to everyone at Children's Hospital of Philadelphia: Dr. Sherry, Lori, Jen, Michelle, Amie, and Tia. You were the ones who helped me learn the skills that I needed to manage and treat my RND. Had it not been for you I would not be writing this book, and I would still be living in fear of my pain's unknowns. You saved my life.

# 1

# *The Gladiator*

○ ○ ○ ○ ○ ○ ○ ○ ○ ○ ○ ○ ○ ○ ○ ○ ○ ○ ○ ○ ○ ○ ○ ○ ○ ○ ○ ○ ○ ○ ○

*Enter at the left ribs. Take a quick left at the T8 vertebra and accel-
erate cranially for 40 centimeters. Upon reaching the scapula, make
a sharp u-turn and descend along the left sternal border. Wait here
for an hour. Repeat.*

For nearly my entire high school career the lancinating pain syndrome
described above has recurred in my body thousands of times without
reprieve. Dozens of doctors have evaluated me, and I have had every blood
test, scan, and procedure imaginable, all without success. The specialists at
the Mayo Clinic called it "idiopathic polyneuropathy." Polyneuropathy—a pain of multiple nerves. Idiopathic—there is no cause or cure, so
we gave it this big name. Instead of using this medical jargon, I prefer a
simpler term, which is now the most frequent word in my vocabu-
lary—ouch!

Everyone's pain is different and hence incomparable, yet through my
own pain I am bonded to others. My pain affects and transforms me, and I
awake enlightened to the First Noble Truth—a heightened sensitivity and
compassion for the suffering of others.

Although having studied the structure and function of nerve cells in AP
Biology, I seldom imagine my own pain in such dehumanizing scientific
terms. Instead, I picture a hostile warrior trapped inside of me. I have
never seen him, but I know he is of the most brutal kind. He is a Roman
Gladiator, fighting to the death. Daily, he struggles to escape, charging at
me with a sharp, glistening spear. He travels throughout my body using

my neurons as his highway, attempting to escape from his prison by ramming a sharp spear into my side.

For much too long I played the role of victim. I watched the Gladiator slowly conquer me; I would close myself up and allow the pain to overtake me. I ceased participating fully in sports and other physical activities because I feared another attack would disable me. Then I had a sudden epiphany: I was getting nowhere playing defense. I had to create my own offense, and so I resumed participating in activities in spite of the pain.

I began to accept pain as a part of who I am. Pain does not define me, nor does it dictate my life. It is a force that teaches me strength and compassion. Yes, there are still days when my unrelenting Comrade pushes me back towards defense. There will always be setbacks, but for the first time since the beginning, I truly feel ahead in the game. I am playing offense, and I'm playing it well!

I don't know whether the Gladiator will ever be loosed from my body, but he no longer controls me. We are partners, working together until we both can be free.

# 2

## *The First Noble Truth*

I wrote "The Gladiator" two years ago in a time of great personal despair and frustration. A senior in high school, I had suffered for over three years with an undiagnosed and unrelenting pain syndrome that had prevented me from enjoying many normal teenage activities. Ultimately, my story will have a happy ending, but it's been a long journey. A journey of pain, sweat, and tears. Was it worth it? I'd say so. Would I want to experience it again? Never. Not in a million years.

About 2500 years ago the Buddha "awakened" to the central problem of existence—human suffering. Buddha's First Noble Truth informs us that all of life is suffering. Every person, regardless of gender, race or age, will experience suffering. Whether it is emotional (fear, sadness, depression) or physical (pain, sickness, injury), suffering is an essential part of being human.

As I dealt with my chronic pain for years, I became more aware of the suffering of others. When someone complained about an illness or acute pain, I listened and tried to show compassion. I must admit that part of my motivation was my desire to learn about a possible cure for myself, but I also believe that I have a heightened awareness of pain in others. After experiencing pain myself and becoming so aware of the suffering of others, I realized that it was impossible to live in this world and not be harmed in some way. Some people get sick, some are in accidents, while I developed chronic pain. The Gladiator was the face I put on my pain to cope with what was happening to my body.

Finally, after a long journey among doctors and medical centers across the country, I have received a proper diagnosis and can at last put a name to the face of the Gladiator. His name is Reflex Neurovascular Dystrophy

(RND). This book is my attempt to alert both physicians and patients to this atypical but devastating syndrome. In three and a half years of dealing with RND, I have seen over twenty different doctors in my effort to find a diagnosis and or cure. Not one of these professionals mentioned RND as a possible diagnosis, and in fact they were largely unaware of the existence of this disorder. I only learned about RND by a random chain of events. It was only by coincidence that my mother spoke to another mother who had a daughter with RND, who could then refer us to the single physician (Dr. David Sherry) who would finally make the correct diagnosis.

So, people need to know what RND is. Plain and simple. I know that if more people (doctors especially) were aware of this condition, there would be fewer people waiting so long to find a diagnosis and treatment. My parents and I wrote a letter to each of the doctors who treated me over the years to inform them of my diagnosis so that they could help people in the future. Already we have heard stories of how these doctors have suggested RND as a diagnosis for other chronic pain sufferers. So, let's get started with the question that is probably on your mind right now:

What is Reflex Neurovascular Dystrophy?

# 3

# *What is Reflex Neurovascular Dystrophy?*

Reflex Neurovascular Dystrophy is a disorder known by many other names: Primary Juvenile Fibromyalgia Syndrome, Chronic Regional Pain Syndrome (CRPS), Amplified Musculoskeletal Pain Syndrome, and Causalgia. RND is related to, and may be a variant of, a more common disorder, Reflex Sympathetic Dystrophy (RSD). Reflex Sympathetic Dystrophy is typically a post-traumatic disorder of the legs or arms accompanied by pain and a bluish discoloration. A new term, RND, is used in several pediatric pain treatment programs to describe the entire group of chronic pain sufferers who do not fit into the classic RSD framework. The mechanisms which cause both conditions are the same, but when a patient presents with symptoms that are unusual (i.e. the pain is not in the typical RSD locations of the extremities), the doctor cannot offer a diagnosis.

First, to understand RND, it is important to understand that pain is a normal and important process that protects our bodies from harm. People with the rare genetic disorder Riley-Day syndrome do not feel pain. This can lead to life threatening injuries, because their bodies are not protected by normal pain signals.

Pain also alerts us to disease and reminds us to get medical attention before the illness progresses too far. However, for a small number of people, these pain signals can persist long after the initial stimulus, injury, or illness is gone. Thus the initially acute pain becomes a chronic condition, which instead of being protective and purposeful becomes aggravating and senseless.

Dr. David Sherry is the Director of Clinical Rheumatology at Children's Hospital of Philadelphia and Professor of Pediatrics at the University of Pennsylvania. He is the world's leading expert on RND. Dr. Sherry developed the new terminology of Reflex Neurovascular Dystrophy to differentiate the pediatric form of RSD from the adult form because the presentation of symptoms, the response to treatment, and the long term prognosis are so very different. While the term RND has not officially been accepted by the International Association for the Study of Pain, it is becoming more widely used in the literature and research on pediatric pain amplification syndromes.

Dr. Sherry's studies show that 80% of RND patients are female. The typical age of an RND patient is between 11-14 years old. It is not as rare as once thought. Dr. Sherry reports that the incidence of RND is two to four children for every 1000.

According to Sherry, RND is a chronic pain cycle stuck in a loop. An exciting factor has to start this loop, however, which may be stress (80%), injury (10-20%), and/or illness. These factors create the initial acute episode of pain. There may be other reasons such as age, genetics, or hormones, but more research needs to be done. After the initial stressor or injury has healed, with RND the pain remains and may even increase.

Sherry has described a possible mechanism by which this process may occur. The pain from the injury travels to the spinal cord and then to the brain as do all pain impulses. But in an RND patient's case, the nerve hits an abnormal reflex in the spinal cord. The pain signal is sent to the brain and to the blood vessels. This causes the blood vessels to constrict, leading to a decrease in oxygen and a build up of acids. The constriction in itself is painful, creating another pain signal to send to the spinal cord. Once it hits the spinal cord, again, the signal is also sent to the blood vessels. Although the injury heals, the pain will remain stuck on this cycle as long as the abnormal reflex is present. RND is a pain amplification syndrome which means that the pain is much more intense than would be expected given the initial cause. It is amplified. (See diagram on following page).

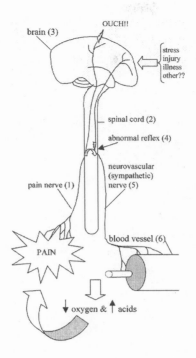

How is the pain signal amplified?

First, look at the figure to see how we normally feel pain. Usually pain is in response to tissue damage, such as stepping on a tack. The damage sends a signal through the pain nerve (1), to the spinal cord (2), then sends the signal up to the brain (3). The brain recognizes the signal as being painful. In RND there is an abnormal short circuit in the spinal cord (4). Therefore, the pain signal not only travels up to the brain, but also goes to the neurovascular nerves (5) that control blood flow through the blood vessels (6). These nerves, however, cause the blood vessels to constrict thus decreasing blood flow. The decreased blood flow deprives the skin, muscles, and bones of oxygen and also leads to a build-up of acid waste products such as lactic acid. This lack of oxygen and acid build-up causes pain. This new pain signal also goes across the abnormal reflex and causes a further decrease in blood flow, thus leading to more pain. Thus, the pain is greatly amplified. RND is a very painful condition.

Diagram and explanation reprinted with permission of Dr. David Sherry.

Most often RND originates in the feet and legs. The next most common location is the hands and arms. RND can be found anywhere in the body, however. It can also migrate from one part of the body to another. Several common signs may occur with RND as well. The skin on the area may turn blue and cold. Also, the affected area experiences a loss of function. For example, a patient may lose the ability to wiggle his or her toes. Another very common symptom is allodynia. Allodynia is a medical term meaning a part of your body is extremely painful to the touch. Sometimes even the wind blowing over one's affected area is enough to cause excruciating pain.

One of the most difficult problems in finding the correct diagnosis for me was that I did not have any of these "classic" symptoms. My pain was primarily located in my ribs and chest wall. My skin did not turn blue or cold; and I did not experience any allodynia. But, I did still have RND. These symptoms are only descriptions of the typical case, but RND can come in many places and forms.

There is no set description of the type of pain one feels with RND. One common attribute of the pain is that it is much more severe and lasts much longer than one would expect from the initiating event. I would describe my pain as "stabbing". Others may feel a hammering, burning, throbbing, etc. No matter what, however, *the pain is real*. RND pain is different for everyone. It can also be constant or, as in my case, intermittent. The fact that my pain migrated and was intermittent was particularly confusing to almost every doctor who examined me.

There is no test for RND, which makes diagnosis difficult. Researchers Murray and Cohen found that the median time to reach a diagnosis of RND is 12 weeks (with a range of 1-130 weeks). Another researcher, Charles Berde, at Harvard Medical School reports from his study of 70 children with RSD that the average time from onset to diagnosis is one year. As a result of such a long interval between the initial pain and the final diagnosis, these children have to endure many unnecessary medical tests, procedures, and medications.

Usually a diagnosis is found from a process of elimination of other testable problems. Even though the doctor, patient, and parents will be

relieved when all of the tests come back normal, it is extren
at the same time. The tests show normal results, but they d
what is causing the pain! When the doctors reported that a
were "normal", my mom had to remind them that it is not "normal" for a
teenage girl to be in pain for over three years. Doctors are sometimes too
dependent on tests to give them the answers. Because of the difference in
presentation from adult pain amplification syndromes, RND is very
under-diagnosed and misdiagnosed in the pediatric population.

Frequently Seen Symptoms of RND

- Pain occurring anywhere on the body

- Pain can be constant or intermittent

- Pain can migrate

- The pain is excruciating and out of proportion to the initial injury

- The affected area can be painful to touch, even a breeze can cause intense pain

- Skin color and temperature changes

- Swelling of the affected area

- Loss of function of the affected area

- Waking from a night's sleep not feeling rested

- Excessive fatigue during the daytime

- Frequent school absences

- Excessive perspiration

- Difficulty focusing and concentrating

- Over-sensitivity to loud noises and large crowds

- Depression

- Poor endurance and low energy levels

- Traditional pain medications have little or no effect in reducing the pain

- Diagnostic tests are normal

# 4

## *Surviving School*

Because the average age of an RND sufferer is between eleven and four-teen, school is an important issue for those who are in chronic pain. And because the average time from onset to diagnosis to treatment is about one year, the student will have a significant amount of their school year affected by their RND. Researchers at Boston's Children's Hospital report that the average number of school days missed due to RND (RSD) is forty days. That is a lot of school and a lot of make-up work. It is possible to have RND and get through high school. I did it, but I had support and cooperation from my teachers and school personnel. If you make accom-modations early on and if you keep the lines of communication open, hopefully you won't have to repeat any part of your middle or high school years.

1. *Communicate with all school personnel about your RND/chronic pain syndrome. Keep them updated on any changes.*

The key to surviving my high school years was communication with all of my teachers, the school administrators, the upper school secretary, and the school nurse. (Don't forget the specialists like music teachers, art teachers, coaches, and PE instructors). When my pain syndrome began and it became clear that it was not going away overnight, my mother arranged a meeting with all of my teachers and administrators. At the beginning of each school year, she would meet with my new teachers and fill them in on my chronic pain syndrome. She would continue to keep them updated by emails. This was especially important when I was trying a new medication because I never knew if I was going to have side effects which would affect my academic performance.

2.   *Ask teachers ahead of time if they are willing to be flexible on due dates for tests and papers or any graded activity.*

Sometimes I was unable to study the night before a test and my teachers would give me an extra day to prepare. I never knew until that night whether I would have a pain flare up, so when it happened I would email them and they were very willing to help me out. I have since realized that these pain flare ups were a response to my increased stress levels right before a big test or exam, but I did not know that at the time.

3.   *Make sure to keep the school secretary in the loop.*

My upper school secretary was very helpful in many ways. She was the main contact person when I was absent. She was helpful in getting my assignments from my teachers. Also, there were many occasions (almost everyday) that I was not able to make it through an entire day of school. Since I had to check in and out with the secretary, it was vital for her to know my situation. I once had a teacher accuse me of skipping class. Yes, this teacher knew all about my pain situation. I had not skipped class, and the records in the office proved that I was at school, but the music teacher had simply overlooked me while taking roll. Out of all of my teachers in high school, this teacher was the only one who did not show compassion and understanding of my pain. Again, having the upper school secretary on my side made a big difference. I didn't get suspended for skipping class!

4.   *Balance the need for accommodations with the need to feel like a normal kid.*

I found that when too many special changes were made for me, the other students were resentful that they did not have the same privileges. Because this is an invisible disease, my classmates were not as understanding of my situation. I tried to keep a "low profile" with my illness. I never bragged when I was allowed to take a test a day late or get an extension on a paper. Usually, no one even noticed. I was on the varsity swim team and I had an agreement with my coach. If my pain became unbearable while swimming laps, I would jump out of the pool and become her assistant for a while until the pain subsided. Then I would get back in the pool and resume my practice. The other members of the team never knew the difference. I was required to attend all practices, just like everyone else, but the coach made special accommodations so that I could be successful and still manage my pain episodes.

5. *If you enter a treatment program during the school year, there will be a school liaison to help you keep up with your work while you are in treatment.*

I was lucky that my treatment occurred after I had finished all of my requirements for graduation. But many of the other patients who were in treatment with me used the educator on the team to help them keep up with their work. The educator also was good at communicating with the school about the patient's condition, progress, and in discussing what she was and wasn't able to complete. It is helpful to have someone prioritize your assignments for you. You may find that it is not necessary for you to do all of the work you are missing, just the most important assignments.

6. *If you do get treatment and are able to return to normal life, please remember to thank everyone who helped you get through this ordeal.*

My teachers did make a difference and I made sure that I told them so. I wanted them to know how much I appreciated their compassion and understanding and it was because of them that I was able to be so successful in high school. Their reply was that I was an inspiration to them.

The Reflex Sympathetic Dystrophy Syndrome Association (RSDSA) has a brochure titled "Helping Children/Youth With RSD/CRPS Succeed in School". They have some excellent ideas on how to modify the classroom for kids who have an amplified pain syndrome. Their guidelines are in accordance with Section 504 of the Rehabilitation Act which prohibits discrimination against individuals with disabilities. This act requires schools to provide equal access to education for kids with disabilities, including chronic pain syndromes. Students may also be eligible for and Individualized Educational Plan (IEP) under the Individuals with Disabilities Education Act (IDEA).

The RSDSA uses the term RSD/CRPS, as they do not recognize RND as a separate form of pediatric RSD. They have collected suggestions from students, parents, educators, and medical professionals. Their recommendations are as follows:

1. Because the slightest bump can cause lasting flare-ups of this very painful syndrome, every effort should be made to see that the child is not exposed to the bumping and jostling of school hallways. The student's desk is each classroom should be positioned away from traffic patterns to avoid inadvertent bumping.

2. Determine whether the student needs ergonomic seating/adjustable desk.

3. Designate another student as a helper who can carry the student's books/belongings during the day, help at lunch, and during the changing of classes.

4. Because students with RSD/CRPS in their upper extremity may have difficulty writing, allow the student to tape record lectures, use a keyboard with a portable word processor, or use another student's notes.

5. Given that RSD/CRPS symptoms can be exasperated by the cold, allow the student to bring a heating pad. Also, guidelines should be developed regarding whether the student should go outside for recess when it is excessively cold; care must be taken to see that the patient has adequate warm clothing, and is kept out of drafts.

6. Allow the student to have an extra set of books at home in addition to school.

7. Permit the student to go to the nurse when needed (may be experiencing a pain flare-up).

8. Permit the student to leave 5 minutes prior to the end of class to avoid the congested hallways.

9. Let the student stretch or take breaks whenever needed.

10. Confer with parents as to whether they wish the student's classmates to be aware of the syndrome.

11. If there is a dress code, the student may need to adapt clothing due to sensitivity to clothing and increased sweating.

12. Special accommodations may be necessary for school field trips, including transportation, medication disbursement, and lodging (if an overnight trip).

13. Ask before touching the student—a simple pat on the back can cause increased pain.

14. Allow a student with RSD/CRPS to sit in a quieter area of the cafeteria if the noise is bothersome; however, do not isolate the student from others.

15. Students with RSD/CRPS are also sensitive to noise and vibrations. Please take this into consideration when fire drills, assemblies, and pep rallies are planned. Allow students to position themselves away from loudspeakers/intercoms—even the classroom bell for beginning and end of class may affect a student with RSD/CRPS.

Reprinted with permission from RSDSA.

# 5

## *What Makes RND Worse?*

### *Illness and Injury*

Everyone gets sick or injured at some point in life; it's a "given". For most people, however, episodes of sickness or injury resolve, and the formerly afflicted areas return to normal. An average teenager may get the flu, for example, and miss a few days of school. Soon, however, she can return to class, sports practice, and everyday life. It is like she was never sick at all (except for the make-up work!) For those with RND, however, this illness or injury can be the main factor in starting the amplified pain cycle, which may keep the afflicted out of regular life for months or even years.

With Reflex Neurovascular Dystrophy, a common initiator of pain comes from either an illness or an injury. Say you break your ankle, for example. The pain from the broken ankle initiates the pain cycle. As the pain signal hits the spinal cord, it generates an abnormal reflex resulting in constriction of the blood vessels. Although the broken bone heals in a few weeks, the pain cycle has already started. The abnormal reflex activates from the pain of the broken bone, and the vicious pain cycle has begun.

Persistent pain in an area that has long since healed is one of the diagnostic factors in determining whether a person has RND. One of the perplexing parts of RND is that while the pain is intense and real, all x-rays, MRIs, bone scans, and other tests are typically normal.

My experience with RND began in a similar fashion. In February, 2003, I was diagnosed with *mycoplasma* pneumonia. I missed two weeks of school, and towards the end of my sickness I developed a severe cough. I could not breathe without coughing. Every fall and every winter I would get pneumonia and end up in the emergency room. My continuous

coughing usually made me hyperventilate. This time, however, my coughing was severe enough to crack one of my ribs.

Eventually my rib healed. But months later the pain from my cracked
rib remained. An x-ray showed that the bone had formed a callus over the
spot where it had cracked. Although the bone was healed, I was paradoxi-
cally in much more pain than when the rib was actually broken.

I was in crippling pain, but my x-ray was normal. My rib shouldn't
have still been hurting. The doctors decided to let it rest and hopefully the
pain would eventually dissipate. Over the next few months, however, I
only found my pain to grow in intensity, frequency, and it began to spread
to other parts of my chest.. This was the beginning of my RND. Unfortunately, I did not find out about what RND was until February of 2006,
and I was not diagnosed until April of that year. But whether I knew about
RND or not, that was what I had, for over 41 months.

## *Stress*

It is well recognized that stress exacerbates all pain, not just RND pain.
But with RND, stress is a key factor (perhaps even more so than in other
chronic pain conditions). RND is one way that our bodies manifest stress.
Some people may show stress by becoming irritable. Others may cry or
even get a stomach ache. Everyone has his way of coping with stressful
times. For those of us with RND, our bodies use stress as fuel for pain. No
one is sure why, exactly. There is not much known at a biological level
about RND. The thing that matters the most, however, is that everything
in your life factors into RND. When I say everything, I mean everything.
Whatever you come into contact with in your daily life can cause stress.

One of the main factors that should be considered about RND is that
stress plays a significant role for 80% of RND patients. Once we understand this concept, we must learn how to reduce stress and manage it in
our lives. Think of the pain as a warning sign. When you feel an increase
in pain, it should be a good sign that you are stressed. Use that sign as a
"stop sign." Sit down, make a list, and evaluate everything in your life.
What is going on lately? Examine your extracurricular activities, friends,

school, and upcoming events. Find the stressor. Then find a way to reduce or eliminate it. Because I may not be consciously aware that I am under stress, my pain has become my indicator of my stress level.

Eliminating stress isn't easy to do. When you evaluate your life, there will be things on the list that you may not want to get rid of. One part of your life you should examine, for example, is your friendships. Although friends can be sources of stress-relief, sometimes you may realize a good friend is actually a huge stressor in your life. What do you do then? Well, that's up to you. But my advice to you is that your health comes first. Maybe you need to get this person out of your life completely. Or, maybe just curtailing your attachment and contact with the person will be enough. If you analyze your friendships, it may become easier to realize that someone in your life is stressful. It may be hard, however, to realize that this stressful person may be increasing your pain. But you need to keep this in mind. Then realize that your health comes first, and help yourself. This becomes a time where you need not worry about the other person, just yourself. I came across this dilemma when I was in the middle of my treatment. A friendship was stressful enough to threaten all the progress that I had made so far in healing, and I realized that my health and healing were more important than a friendship that caused me actual physical pain.

Wanting to please people and be overly willing and nice are personality traits commonly found in RND patients. But this kind of personality can create a lot of stress. It is not easy to please people all the time. In fact it is impossible. And when you are too focused on making everyone else happy, you forget about what makes you happy.

Learning to take care of myself is one of the most valuable lessons I have discovered through my experience with RND. I know that I can sit here and tell you about what I have experienced, but I also know that it is not easy to accept my advice if you have not realized these lessons first hand. If you have RND, your body is giving you the perfect opportunity to directly and intimately explore the need to respect your body.

Obviously it is impossible in our fast paced American lives to avoid stress. In fact, RND is much more likely to be found in American adolescents because of the huge amounts of energy (and accompanying stress) it takes to keep up with our society.

For the past three and a half years, I did not know that I had RND and therefore did not realize the direct influence of stress on my pain. Had I known, however, I do not think that I would have been able to reduce much stress in my life nonetheless. I was in high school. I had to deal with the pressures of puberty, social scenes, and the well-known pressure of getting into college. In order to get into my first choice of colleges I had to take challenging courses, keep up my grades, and juggle all of my extracurricular activities. Eliminating these stressors was out of the question.

So, had I been concerned with keeping stress to a minimum in my life at that time, I would have then needed to re-evaluate the things in my life that I could change. Maybe I could have changed the types of activities in which I was participating to ones I purely enjoyed. Maybe I could have learned how to better manage my friendships and stay clear of negative people. Obviously it is too late to change the past, but my point is that there are some things that cannot be eliminated. I understand that other people may have different priorities than these, but sometimes the priorities will be contributing to your RND and causing stress. There are always stressors that can be reduced, however. Find those, and use that knowledge to your advantage.

Another way to reduce stress is to allow yourself to have "down time" every day. I have found that when I am constantly on the go, maybe for days at a time, my pain increases. No matter whether the activities I fill my days with are stressful or not, being busy all the time is stressful. So, try to devote a certain amount of "chill time" to each day. My goal is to allow two hours every day. Allowing down time will keep you from over committing to too many activities. It will help you to budget your time and really ask yourself what you want the most. Make this a high priority in your daily life.

Here are two tips for reducing the amount of activities in your life and enjoying what you do:

1. Ask yourself before committing: "Is this what I *really* want?" If you cannot honestly answer "I want this", then do not feel compelled to commit.

2. Allow yourself to say "no" to people without giving excuses. A simple "no, I'm sorry I can't" will suffice. If you say, "No, I can't because ..." and supply some reason, people find ways to get around the excuse. If people can't take a simple "no", then that is their problem!

Because RND sufferers tend to be "people pleasers", these two ideas do not come naturally. Therefore, you will have to practice these everyday until they become automatic. Write out these statements on index cards and put them where you can read them several times a day. I put them by my phone so when co-workers call to ask me to work overtime to cover their shifts, I can say, "No, I'm sorry. I can't." without feeling guilty.

You can't always control events around you, but you can control your response to them. Here are some important points which will make it easier for you to have a healthy response to stressful situations.

1. Make daily goals that are realistic and attainable.

2. Remember the goal is progress, not perfection.

3. Talk to friends, be with people. Don't isolate yourself.

4. Have some down time each day for yourself, without isolating yourself too much.

5. Give yourself an occasional treat.

6. Play relaxing music, especially right before bed.

7. Get rid of your "toxic" friends. Surround yourself with friends who bring out your best qualities.

8. If you feel like you are totally consumed by your pain, reach out and help someone else. It will help take the focus off of your pain for a little while.

9. Take care of your personal appearance. Good grooming/hygiene are very important.

10. Make a list of things that you do well and do them on a regular basis.

11. Make a list of your best qualities. Get input from family and friends. Post it where you can see it everyday.

12. Laugh, watch funny movies. Stay away from drama!

13. Eat a healthy and well balanced diet.

14. Get plenty of sleep, 8-10 hours. Keep a regular bedtime and wake-up time.

15. Drink plenty of water. Stay hydrated. Your brain and your muscles will function better. (I am a strong advocate of this).

16. Exercise. Take the stairs instead of the elevator.

17. Simplify your life. Reduce your schedules and activities. Even getting rid of clutter will make you feel better.

While living in chronic pain for nearly four years without a diagnosis, I had many fears. The pain took on a life of its own and the uncertainty of it caused much anxiety and fear, which in turn led to more stress. Here are the things that I feared the most:

- *Not waking up.*

  I had no idea what was wrong with me. The pain was so intense that I thought I must have some horrible disease and I was going to die.

- *Waking up and still being in pain.*

  Every night when I went to sleep, I had to deal with the fear that tomorrow would be yet another day like today, living in chronic pain with no end in sight.

- *Stumping another doctor.*

  I was afraid that I would run out of doctors. Where would I go next if this doctor couldn't cure me?

- *Lost and damaged relationships.*

  I lost good friends because of my pain. No one understood what I was going through on a day to day basis. It happened many times and I couldn't bear to lose any more ties.

- *Causing future pain.*

  If I was feeling good and trying to keep up with normal activities, I knew I would pay for it the next several days with increased pain. It was fun to roller skate for an afternoon, but I always feared the pain it would cause the following day. I already had enough pain.

- *Having a poor quality of life forever.*

  Nothing was helping. It seemed like only a miracle could save me from living my life in chronic pain forever.

- *Is it all in my head?*

  People and doctors who don't believe you put this idea in your head. I often would doubt myself when others doubted my pain. But I had to remind myself that MY PAIN IS REAL.

- *Missing out on life.*

  My high school years were passing by very quickly and I was missing out on many fun activities. I was afraid that I wouldn't have any fond recollections of high school, just memories of the pain. After treatment and I went to college, my doctor told me that there would be times when I would have to put my studying aside. She told me that I need to make up for the fun I missed in high school.

# 6

## *What Makes RND Better?*

### *Treatment*

You now understand what Reflex Neurovascular Dystrophy is and what causes it. But now you're probably wondering, "How do I get rid of RND?"

Dr. David Sherry has developed a treatment program focused on eliminating RND pain and teaching the patients about the complexities of the syndrome. His inspiration comes from the work of two other physicians, Virgil Hanson and Bram Bernstein. Dr. Sherry's treatment program has an intense focus on physical and occupational therapies. "There are few studies of long-term outcome. In one study where the children were treated with an intense exercise program, 92% reached full function at the end of two weeks of treatment and 88% were pain free after an average of five years" (Sherry). The success rates are primarily based on anecdotal evidence, and physician observations suggest that children and adolescents have a much higher recovery rate than adults with similar pain syndromes.

Most patients are taken off all medications, with the exception of antidepressants and some sleep medicine. All other pain medications interfere with retraining the nerve pathways. Occasionally, the patient will need to be admitted as an overnight patient at the hospital, but this is not usually the case. Some reasons for in-patient treatment are to monitor the patient when she is weaning off medicines or to help break the patient's dependency on the mother. Typically, one only needs to come for the day. The average patient spends three to four weeks in the program, attending Monday through Friday sessions of therapy from 9:00 am to 4:00 pm. The patients go home with an exercise program to complete on the weekends.

Parents normally are not allowed to visit their children during the treatment day and are not permitted to attend therapy sessions, as it is necessary for the patients to separate from their parents. This is because most RND patients have been out of school for long periods of time, and the rule is a way to get them back into a school feeling.

This treatment program exemplifies the adage "no pain, no gain." Normally, one would associate this motto with sports training to become a better athlete. But when applied to RND, it means that if an activity increases your pain, then do it more. The theory with this treatment is that when you are increasing pain, you are also increasing blood flow to the nerve endings in that area. Your body is sending you a pain signal in an effort to keep you from completing this action. For example, when you try to walk on your foot, your body will send pain signals so that you will stop walking on the hurt foot. To treat RND, you must walk on your foot no matter how much it hurts to show your body that even though it is sending pain signals, you must not keep yourself from walking. Such a process retrains the nerves and eventually the pain signals will stop. You will have to rethink how you process pain. In this treatment program, when you are taught that if an action causes you to hurt, it doesn't mean it will cause you harm or injury.

RND treatment is divided into two components. Phase I is the time spent in the hospital participating in the daily therapy sessions. Phase II occurs once you return home, and involves regaining your normal life. These phases will now be described in more detail.

# PHASE I

Phase I takes place at the hospital. As an RND patient in the day hospital, you will participate in a variety of therapies for several hours each day. The following explanation is from my personal experience as a patient in an RND treatment program. There are many more activities than the ones I will describe, and each treatment program is adapted to each patient's specific needs. I have listed some of the basic activities that everyone must do as part of treatment. But your treatment program will be tailored to your individual pain and interests, so you will have some different exercises as well.

The typical activities I will describe are part of Dr. David Sherry's treatment program at the Children's Hospital of Philadelphia (CHOP). There are only a few RND centers in the country that treat RND according to Dr. Sherry's protocol. (These centers are listed in the additional resources section of this book.) These centers use a team approach that includes a pediatric rheumatologist or other physician, physical and occupational therapists, psychologist, a school liaison, a social worker, and others as deemed necessary for each patient's individual treatment plan, (e.g., at CHOP they have a music therapist). The goal of therapy in Phase I is for function to return by the end of the 3-4 week program. The pain will normally decrease, but will take much longer to go away completely.

## Physical Therapy

You will meet with the physical therapist for one on one treatment. This is where you will spend most of your time, doing physical therapy (PT) exercises, which are highly aerobic. You will break a sweat for sure in PT. Physical therapy is especially hard for RND patients because they have curtailed their normal activities for an extended period of time due to their pain. The endurance exercises are designed specifically for each patient. Many of these activities are designed to allow you to return to specific sports that you used to play before RND.

In order to keep your focus on your function and not your level of pain, you will be required to complete a set of timed tasks every day. The objective is to beat your time from the day before until you can consistently achieve the time it takes an average healthy person your age to complete the task. You will have to repeat the activity until you do so. This ensures that you will continue to get better each day and not suffer any setbacks if you don't feel well or if your pain fluctuates while in the program. The most commonly dreaded timed activities are the animal walks. Each day you must walk a certain distance like a crab, a 3-legged puppy, a duck, an inch worm, and a frog. And each day you must cover this distance in less time than the day before. Other activities include a 90 ft sprint, a wheelbarrow pull, step ups, and arm step ups.

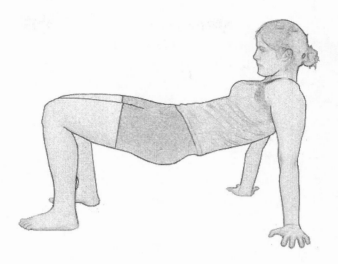

Crab Walk

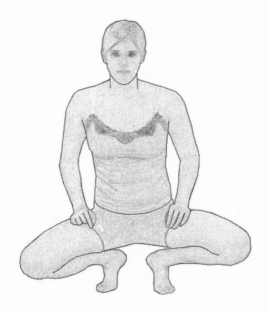

Duck Walk

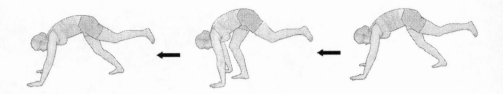

3-Legged Puppy

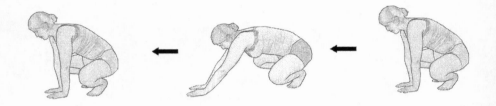

Frog Walk

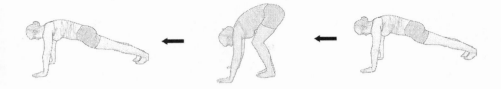

Inch Worm Walk

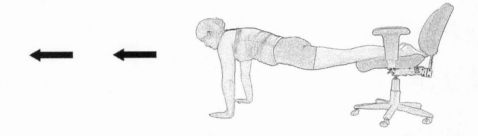

Wheelbarrow Pull

The wheelbarrow pull is 100 ft. Imagine you are the "wheelbarrow" in a wheelbarrow race with your friend, only your friend is instead a chair with wheels on it. So, in essence you must pull yourself with your arms 100 ft with your legs up in a chair. Be aware; the chair tips easily, but as long as you keep your stomach tightened it will tip less. This is a great exercise for your arms and abdominal muscles.

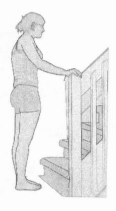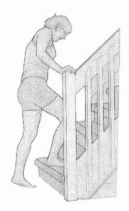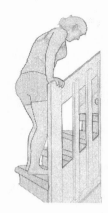

## Step-Ups

Step-ups are just like in an aerobic class. Left foot up, right foot up. Left foot down, right foot down. Up, up, down, down. You must do this forty times. Then, you will repeat this, stepping up and down with your right foot first instead of the left. Don't forget that you still must beat your times from the previous day.

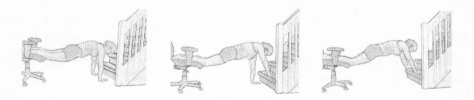

## Arm Step-Ups

Arm step-ups are very similar to the leg step-ups. The only catch is that you are in the same wheelbarrow stance. You must then move your arms like your legs did in the regular step ups. These were my least favorite by far of any timed activity.

Once per week everyone must complete an endurance test called "The Bruce" (after its creator). This is a treadmill test where each three minutes the incline and speed increase. So at about fifteen minutes, you are sprinting uphill.

These are the standard activities for everyone. But as I said earlier, your program will be tailored to your individual needs. If RND is in your foot, then you will have more lower extremity exercises like walking, running, jumping, etc.

In the evenings and on weekends, you will be encouraged to remain active. Even though it was painful to just walk, my mother made sure that we saw all of the tourist spots in Philadelphia. Keeping active also helps keep your mind off of your sore muscles and RND pain.

## Occupational Therapy

Occupational therapy (OT) is centered on helping you return to everyday activities such as cooking, going to the bathroom, etc. There are fewer timed activities in OT. Some examples of timed OT exercises are stepping in and out of a bathtub as many times as possible in thirty seconds or carrying an 11 lb. box and squatting to put it on and lift it off the floor.

In some cases, such as mine, not much needs to be improved on daily activity ability. So, we focused mainly on desensitization. As I described in the "What is RND?" section, allodynia is the symptom of being painful to touch. Desensitizing attacks this problem. How? By touching the painful area with unpleasant surfaces. This can include vibration, massage, heat, ice, sand, etc. Any sort of direct contact with the skin to cause pain is desensitization. It sounds like cruel and unusual punishment, but it eventually helps with the overall treatment.

You may not find that you have allodynia currently and it is possible to have RND without this symptom. I did not experience allodynia for the three and a half years I endured RND. When I got to CHOP and began treatment, however, I developed allodynia. This new symptom was actually a good sign because it meant that the nerves were beginning to link up with the blood vessels, and once I attacked the allodynia I would get better. It was eerie to have a sensitive-to-touch area on my body, but by massaging the area and treating it with vibrations, the allodynia disappeared along with the RND.

## Pool Therapy

Pool therapy is a way to break up the schedule with something different. Pool therapy usually consists of activities like water aerobics. This kind of therapy is different from land based exercises because the water makes you more buoyant and takes pressure off of joints and sore areas. The effect of this will be increased mobility. Furthermore, water provides resistance which helps strengthen muscles. Since I am a swimmer, the team tried to provide extra pool therapy times for me.

Pool therapy is also a time to focus on desensitization. With allodynia even air hurts the skin, so water hurts as well. Patients are forced to put the affected body part in the water to help attack the allodynia. Like I said, it sounds cruel. But, sometimes you have to do what you have to do. This is also a form of occupational therapy because when you overcome the allodynia you can return to daily functioning activities such as bathing and washing your hair.

## Music Therapy

Music therapy is a time to take a break from the fast-paced physical activity. Generally you meet with a trained music therapist who is part of the treatment team once or twice per week. Through music you learn relaxation techniques for reducing stress. This also helps with muscle relaxation and pain reduction. Music therapy can also be used as a way for you to express your feelings about pain. This was one of my favorite times of the week and one of the few activities I actually looked forward to!

## Talk Time

"Talk Time" is time set aside to meet with the RND team's psychologist. Typically you meet twice a week, for an hour at a time (and more, as needed), to help you cope with the intense emotional aspects of the treatment program. This session is a good time to examine the circumstances in your life that may be causing stress and to learn how you can better handle these situations. An additional benefit of learning how to reduce stressful situations is that it makes you feel more in charge of your life. When you feel empowered and have some control over your life you no longer are a "victim" of chronic pain. This is an important part of your recovery as well.

Often there are other psychological factors which may be contributing to your RND, such as depression, anxiety, and eating disorders. You may need help dealing with some personality traits which also go along with RND, such as perfectionism, control needs, and people-pleasing. The psychologist can meet with other family members in order to help you make the transition from the hospital to the home environment. The psychologist can also help you find a mental health professional near your home to provide further assistance and support for you and your family. RND is a disorder which affects the entire family. It is important to change the family's behaviors and responses to RND pain.

I have some general guidelines about what to expect with the treatment. These tips are not meant to alarm you, but to let you know what is normal. First, about Day Three you will be the sorest. Don't worry; the sore muscles will go away. Just remember to stretch a lot. I cannot emphasize that enough. Stretching will help decrease muscle soreness, and it will also help reduce the chance of injury.

The second week of treatment is commonly the worst. The pain might get worse before it gets better. Also by the second week, your body will be physically exhausted and your mind will be emotionally worn out. But keep on going. You will find that you are stronger than you think you are.

You will find yourself doing so much exercise that you will be pushed to tears. It is okay, let them go. You also may feel like vomiting, and you may vomit. I just want you to have a warning that it will be this hard. Don't be scared though, you can do it. And if you get through this part, you will be well on your way to being pain free! What could be a better reward?

Dismissal from the program comes once the team feels that you have a good grasp on what you need to do to continue treatment. You must have a comprehensive understanding of what RND is and what aggravates it, especially stress. I have found that this was one of the hardest parts of the treatment program. Once you understand RND fully, then your pain will be much easier to manage and diminish.

It is not unusual to be released before all pain has disappeared, however. In fact, often an increase in pain can be seen right before dismissal from the program. This is because of the anxiety that comes with knowing you will be on your own to treat the pain once released. I definitely saw an increase in my pain a few days before I was released. They assured me that it was common. I was scared that I would not be able to handle the treatment at home by myself and that since my pain was not completely gone that it would return.

You will find that after three or four weeks of intensive therapy you have regained your strength, your endurance, and your agility. If you continue to do what your team tells you once you go home, your pain will continue to wane. When you have been dismissed from the hospital, you are ready to begin Phase II, which is a longer and much different process than Phase I.

# PHASE II

When you are dismissed from the hospital you will be given a home exercise program to continue every day. But Phase II encompasses much more than a continuation of exercise on your own. This is the time to put into effect the stress reduction tools you gained while at the hospital. This is the time to learn how to take care of your needs first.

At this point you need to try to get back into a completely normal routine. Do the things you used to do. Don't let your pain stop you now. BE NORMAL AGAIN. Rediscover the "you" that may have been lost during your battle with RND. And remember, this is the time to reduce the stressors in your life.

Phase II is much longer than Phase I. You get to decide when you are finished with this phase. But you may find that you are never finished. This may be something you need to keep tabs on for the rest of your life. About 30% of RND patients have a relapse and a majority of those occur within six months of treatment. Half of those are able to catch it early and cure it at home with an exercise program. The key is early awareness and starting treatment as soon as possible. The tricky part, however, is recognizing new pain as RND. Many relapses occur in different parts of the body. Half of those with relapses say the pain is the same and half say the pain is much different from their first episode of RND. Not all new pain will turn out to be RND, but you should think of this as a possible source, especially if the pain is out of proportion to the initiating event.

You may decide that once your pain is completely gone that you can forget about all of the RND exercises. For me, I will take what I have learned and apply it to every day for the rest of my life. Phase II never will end for me. I will continue to manage my stress levels and try to exercise when I can. I may not exercise every day, but I know how to handle my pain and balance my need for exercise along with the other areas of my life.

But again, this is up to you. At this point in treatment you have learned how to effectively manage your life. At this point it's a balancing act. But you have trained long and hard and are now a pro.

Suggestions for the family when the RND patient returns home after treatment:

- Learn everything you can about Reflex Neurovascular Dystrophy.

- Don't focus on my pain.

- Don't ask me how my pain is. If I need to, I will tell you.

- Don't rearrange the family's schedules, plans, or activities because of my RND.

- Don't reward me when I am in pain. If you give me extra attention or treats when I am in pain, you will just reinforce my pain.

- Listen to me when I need to talk, but don't offer solutions to problems unless I ask. Let me try to figure things out for myself.

- Exercise with me. It gets lonely and boring exercising by myself everyday.

- Let me be a normal kid. I have missed a lot of life, so I have some catching up to do.

# 7

## *Success in this Program*

What is your definition of success? For most people, it means to achieve a goal, to accomplish something that they set out to do. A common desire for those who enter an RND treatment program is to be successful by eliminating their pain by the end of their treatment.

"I wish to leave treatment with absolutely no pain." That is a common objective among patients. As described in the treatment section a few pages earlier, Phase II continues long after you leave the hospital and the PT program. When you leave the hospital after Phase I, your pain most likely will not be completely gone. The primary goal of Phase I of treatment is to regain your function. Success at that point should be measured by how you are able to function compared to other kids your age. You want to become normal again, so that is the criterion you should use for success at the end of Phase I.

My advice is to not get your hopes set on complete pain relief at this stage of the game. A complete cure is too much to ask for after only a few weeks of treatment. Remember, your pain has been with you for much longer than three or four weeks. I could not expect nearly four years of chronic pain to disappear after four weeks of treatment. That would not be a realistic goal and I would just be setting myself up for failure. If you set your hopes too high and are let down when some pain still remains, you will be inclined to think that the treatment was a failure. This kind of thinking could cause you to lose all motivation and the pain may very well come back in full force.

What if your pain gets significantly better but never completely goes away? Would you consider that a success or a failure? This is what happened to me, and I consider myself to be extremely successful. When I realized that it is possible that my pain won't go away completely, I stepped back and reevaluated how far I had come. I reworked my goal into something much more hopeful. I measured my success by the degree to which I had been able to return to an active, healthy, and completely normal life. By recognizing the accomplishment of these goals, I consider myself a success of the treatment. I am able to function normally every day, and I am back to feeling and acting like my old self in spirit. That's all that one could really ask for, right?

Success isn't necessarily how far you get, but rather it is how far you have come. Just keep this in mind when you are healing: the pain will get better and your function will return. Measure success in terms of this statement, and even if you aren't 100% pain free, you stand the chance of becoming 100% successful. Progress, not perfection, is your goal.

*Success isn't necessarily how far you get,*
*But rather it is how far you have come.*

# 8

## *Moving On: You Can't Just Forget*

Now you are at the point where you have been through treatment and you are ready to get on with your life. At this stage of writing I have been out of Phase I for six months. I have more or less started a new way of life, with new priorities and coping strategies to better deal with flare ups of pain. Six months out of Phase I, I still do have some pain. I am not one hundred percent cured, and I don't know if I ever will be. I am, however, *significantly* better. The pain no longer controls my life. I know what it is and how to deal with it when it does occasionally recur. At this point my pain serves merely as a reminder of the past.

During a recent flare up of my RND, I got extremely depressed. I let myself twist my definition of "success" into being completely pain free. Since I was not pain free, I began to feel that the program had not worked. This depression was due not only to the fact that my pain was still present, but also because I felt so utterly alone. I know that I am not; there are others who have RND and go through the same thing that I do in dealing with the illness, yet I wanted more than anything to have a best friend who shared it with me. I wished so badly that I knew someone who was being treated with RND that went to school with me and who I talked to every day. I began to realize that since I am now in college, none of the people I will meet will know about this part of my past. That thought made me feel even more alone than I had felt in high school, because in high school all my friends and teachers watched me deal with the RND and had a better idea of what I was coping with. At college, no one knew or had seen me deal with RND at my worst times.

While I was in my depressed state, my mom said something to me that resonated, and it made me write this chapter in the book. I had explained to her that even the people who I knew with RND and those I met in treatment really weren't enthusiastic about keeping in contact with me and talking to me about our pain. Then I told her that because of this lack of enthusiasm to keep in touch, I had not been able to make a good friend with whom I could talk whenever I was feeling down about my RND. My mom responded, "Maybe they just want to forget."

And here is my piece of wisdom for this chapter: you can't just forget. As much as you want to say that the RND is a small part of your life and you can be treated and move on, it is impossible to forget the pain you suffered and the treatment you endured. You cannot forget that RND is a part of you. Imagine your life as a book and each new experience as a chapter. RND would constitute a chapter in this book. But the book is not closed, and you cannot go back and delete the chapter because the memories do not please you.

Rather, you must use your unpleasant memories as fuel for your journey. You must take what you can from your experience and apply it to your outlook on life every day. I believe that we can learn something valuable from every life experience. How can you not learn something, anything, from dealing with some of the worst pain you may have ever felt in your life? If you treat this chapter of RND in your life rather as a "closed book" and try to forget about your battle with RND, then every bit of your experience was a waste of time, energy, and sorrow.

A doctor that I have seen regularly for over a year refers to herself as a "Mind-Body Specialist." She is an MD, yet she no longer works in the traditional doctor's office. Dr. Diane Morrow deals with patients who suffer from a variety of chronic conditions. She practices a holistic form of medicine, "Mind Body Medicine" with the philosophy that you must listen to your body because it tells you important information. For example, my body will send RND pain signals when I am stressed. She teaches me how to read my physical body reactions and interpret them into a way to live well. It is a holistic approach, and I have found her philosophy very valuable in helping me live a better and healthier life.

The reason I mention Dr. Morrow in this chapter is to further empha-size the point that you must learn from your experience, and secondly to remind you that you can't do this alone. Do not compartmentalize your RND and box it off once you have been treated. Listen to your body and it may tell you why you may have become a victim of RND. If you listen and learn, you can then go on to teach others what you have learned from your experience. Not only will you learn about how to manage your RND, but you will learn life long lessons. But I beg you, do not try to forget. If you forget your past experiences, the pain will probably come back. You will begin to slip into your old ways by not thinking about RND and how you can prevent it, and the pain may creep up on you. And then, you truly have learned nothing, not even the basic lesson of the physical therapy treatment which is to learn how to control and prevent future pain. And then what really is the point in everything you went through before if you end up back at the beginning?

So, if you use your RND to self analyze, you will learn lessons which you can apply to your life. Doing so will help you grow and mature, it will teach others, and it will remind you of RND so that you do not slip back into the endless pain cycle. Writing this book is what I have done to remember my pain. I have learned very valuable lessons from my experi-ence with RND, and it would have been a waste if I had not taken this opportunity to share what I have learned with others.

---

*Use your unpleasant memories*
*As fuel for your journey.*

---

# 9

## *I Know It's Frustrating*

I know it's frustrating having chronic pain. It's even more exasperating when you don't have a diagnosis. I can't even begin to count how many tears were shed throughout my battle with RND. Nor can I count how many times I walked out of the doctor's office feeling that the doctors had no idea what was wrong with me.

A problem that I ran across numerous times was the fact that doctors are too specialized. They have to be; the body is so complex that knowing it so thoroughly is practically impossible. So, I basically made the rounds to a variety of specialists to test each of my major organ systems.

Unfortunately, each time I saw a doctor, he usually seemed unable to look outside of his field. For example, because I went to see a neurologist, she had to try to find what was wrong with me neurologically. When I saw a gastroenterologist; he tried to make my pain the result of some sort of GI problem. I was diagnosed with everything from post-herpetic neuralgia to constipation!

I don't blame any of these doctors for thinking this way. They went to years of school to become experts in their fields. It only makes sense that they would try to find my answer from their certain area of expertise. I guess what made it wearisome was the fact that these doctors would search and search but still come up with nothing. Sometimes they would force a diagnosis on me which I knew was incorrect, but they were frustrated too.

Just keep all of this in mind. They want to find the solution too! They really do. Most doctors are not familiar with the diagnosis of RND. They know a lot about their specialties, however, and they will do everything they can within their knowledge to figure out the answer. Unfortunately,

51

they often are unable to look outside their field of expertise, and this can be discouraging when you are looking for a diagnosis.

*I know having a doctor believe your problem fits into their specialty is frustrating.*

I was the most frustrated when a doctor actually gave up on me. I had never imagined a patient going to a doctor who would actually give up after exhausting all of his options. But it happened many times. I'm sure it's frustrating for them to be stumped and have to turn a patient away. I was so discouraged when the medical professionals gave up trying to find a diagnosis and a cure for my pain.

At one point I saw a pain specialist, trained in anesthesiology. He tried two very invasive procedures, which included injecting my spine with steroids. All I wanted for Christmas that year was to be pain free on Christmas Day. It didn't happen. The spinal procedure only gave me twenty four hours of pain relief and by Christmas Eve the pain had returned.

The pain specialist tried everything he could think of. He prescribed several medications, all of which barely masked the pain. On my last visit to him he recommended trying capsaicin cream. I tried it and it burned like hell! This is when I realized that he had given up on my pain and I had given up on him. Because he was a pain specialist, I had such high hopes. When he ran out of ideas I was crushed.

*I know having a doctor give up on you is frustrating.*

Another frustrating part of my pain journey was the variety of medications I was prescribed. Every doctor I saw wanted to give me a new prescription. At one point I was taking twelve pills a day (plus Tylenol).

Before I developed RND, I rarely needed to take any medicines. I rarely took Tylenol either. I don't like medicines. It's not that I don't believe in them, but I feel that often they can end up doing more harm than helping. Sometimes the side effects outweigh the benefits. I have always been in favor of letting the problem fix itself (like letting the headache go away on its own rather than taking pain killers).

Shortly after my RND began, however, all of that went out the window. I was desperate for any relief. I carried Tylenol and Ibuprofen with me everywhere I went. I was okay with that. But what I hated most was that every time I went to the doctor, he wanted to prescribe a new medication to alleviate the pain. It was so frustrating knowing that the next step was always to try a new medicine. Once the doctor would recommend starting a new medicine, I would have to wean off of my current medicines before starting the new one. He would then tell me it would take several weeks/months to determine if it was going to be effective or not. Next he would run down the list of side effects. Sometimes more medicines were added to counteract the side effects of the new medication.

I was tolerant at first, when I still had hope that medication would be the answer. But every time I tried a new medicine, the only part of it that worked was the side effects. None of the medicines I tried reduced my chronic pain by any significant amount. (As I would later find out, medicines do not normally help RND pain).The common side effect of all the medications was drowsiness. Couple that with not sleeping well from the pain, and eventually I couldn't make it through the day without a nap. I would wake up for school in the morning, and the only way I could get out of bed was by knowing I could come home from school and take a nap. I started the day with a cup of strong coffee. That was usually enough to get me to school and part way through my first class. By mid-morning I would need another caffeine boost. I was miserable, and it made me dislike medicines even more.

*I know taking medicines, coping with side effects, and having little or no relief is frustrating.*

Some people like to call RND the "invisible illness." That's an accurate description of this disorder. It is so hard to suffer every day and not have obvious signs of the suffering. I had no external signs of illness or injury, no visible proof that I was in pain. My pain was invisible to my friends, teachers, family, doctors, everyone! Sometimes I wished that I were on crutches or in a cast so that people could understand that there actually was something wrong with me. That way others would understand why I missed so much school or why I could only walk around the track instead of run. I am sure there were people who did not believe that I was in pain.

*I know having an "invisible" ailment is frustrating.*

# 10

## *Parenting a Child with RND*

By: Jeanine Elster

Although I have been through the three and a half years of chronic pain with Elizabeth, my journey has been a different one. My perspective as a parent of a child/teen with RND is different from the pain sufferer's perspective. I want to take a few moments to tell you how I managed to get through these years with Elizabeth and her pain and what I learned along the way.

*The most important thing I did for Elizabeth was that I never gave up trying to find a cure for her pain.* At some point after numerous doctors and tests I did give up trying to find the cause of her pain, and I would have just settled for finding anything that would stop her pain for good.

We traveled to over twenty doctors covering fifteen different specialties in three states before we found an answer. Each and every doctor thought that they knew the cause and the cure. Every time she went to the doctor, they had a new medication for her to try. Each one told her that it would take at least 6 weeks or longer for her to know if the new medication would work or not. She endured dozens of blood tests, radiological procedures, injections in her spine and ribs, physical therapy, nuclear scans, etc. One recurring thought was that she was suffering from post-herpetic neuralgia from an outbreak of shingles she had at age ten. Many of the medications she tried were for this specific condition. The most common mixture of meds included an antidepressant, an anti-seizure medication, and an anti-inflammatory. Within each of these categories of drugs, she tried many different medications. This combination, however, did take the edge off her pain and make it tolerable most of the time. We saved traditional pain medications, such as narcotics, for emergencies only.

Elizabeth saw medical experts at Wake Forest Medical Center, the Pediatric Pain Clinic at Duke University, the Adolescent Diagnostic and Referral Clinic at the Mayo Clinic in Rochester, Minnesota, and finally the RND team at the Children's Hospital of Philadelphia. The twenty+ doctors she saw included:

- Pediatricians (2)

- Adolescent specialists (2)

- Neurologist

- Orthopedist

- Allergy/Immunologist

- Pulmonologist

- Urologist

- Gynecologist

- Gastroenterologists (2)

- Physiatrist

- Anesthesiologists/Pain

- Management Specialists (2)

- Rheumatologists (2)

- Psychiatrist/Psychologist (3)

- Mind Body Physician

- Internist/Family Practice

- Occupational Therapist

- Physical Therapists (3)

Some of the medications she tried included:

- Antidepressants

- Anti-seizure medications

- Anti-inflammatories

- Steroids

- Muscle relaxants

- Beta blockers

- COX-2 inhibitors

- Narcotics (for emergencies)

- Advil/Tylenol

- Antiviral medications

- Hormones

- Antibiotics (for repeated mycoplasma pneumonias)

- Tramadol

I spent hours and hours researching her problem on the Internet. One day I came across RSD and asked my physician husband if Elizabeth could possibly have that disorder. He dismissed it quickly because her symptoms did not fit the typical profile of a person with RSD. It was over a year later that by chance I stumbled upon RND and Dr. Sherry.

Elizabeth was a real trooper throughout this ordeal. She tolerated my continual search and tried my sometimes wacky ideas. When she would get discouraged, I always had a new plan, a new idea to try. Sometimes I would go to the drugstore and just look on every shelf for some new kind of pain reliever that she hadn't tried yet. Here are some of the "cures" I came up with:

- Acupuncture

- Meditation/hypnosis

- Relaxation therapy

- Deep tissue massage

- Vitamins/mineral supplements

- Natural oils to rub on the spots that hurt

- Biofeedback

- Yoga/Pilates

- Heat packs/cold packs

- TENS unit

- Creams/ointments

- Steroid injections

- Wearing loose clothing, no tight undergarments around the painful area

- Magnetic wrist band, like those worn for motion sickness

- Numerous dietary changes/restrictions

- Laxatives (the doctors at Duke told us the pain was from constipation)

- Increasing water intake

- Room air purifier (this did help her coughing spells)

We even tried "total denial" that the pain even existed, but that didn't work either. But all of these attempts to find a cure continued to give Elizabeth hope and reassurance that I had not given up.

Besides telling you as a parent or loved one to never give up hope, the other important piece of advice I have is to *keep networking and talking about the problem to everyone you know,* (or to anyone who will listen!). This is how I found the answer and the cure for Elizabeth's pain.

One day Elizabeth complained of lower back pain after running on the treadmill at the YMCA. Her back pain persisted for several days and continued to get worse. Fearing that her rib pain had migrated to her lower back, we again investigated. Her internist ordered an MRI of her spine. My husband and I thought that maybe we would finally see something that would point to the cause of her pain.

I remembered that the son of a friend of mine had back problems several years ago, so I called Susanna to ask her what she did for her son's back, which doctor treated him, and who his physical therapist was. We decided that it had been too long since we had talked and we made plans to meet for lunch the next day. (Later it was determined that Elizabeth did not have a defect in her spine, but the fact that it was mentioned led me to make the phone call and reconnect with an old friend).

It had been over three years since I had talked to Susanna, as she did not know about Elizabeth's chronic pain syndrome. I told her the whole story from the beginning and all that we had been through trying to find an answer. I will never forget the moment when she looked across the table and said, "I have a friend whose daughter had exactly the same thing." I tried not to get my hopes up, but agreed to let her call the friend and ask if she would share her story with me. The next day I spoke to the friend, Debbie, and the similarities between her daughter Elysia's pain and my Elizabeth's pain were too close to be a coincidence. I had never met anyone who could even begin to relate to our situation. I got the name of the doctor who diagnosed and cured her and found him on the internet. I researched this new disorder, RND, and the more I found out about it, the more hopeful I was that this was the answer we had been searching for.

I made an appointment for Elizabeth to see Dr. David Sherry, a pediatric rheumatologist at the Children's Hospital of Philadelphia (CHOP) who specializes in the treatment of RND. On April 17, 2006 Elizabeth and I flew to Philadelphia for the day and spent over an hour with Dr.

Sherry. While he confirmed the diagnosis of RND, I was still afraid to get my hopes up. Every doctor Elizabeth had ever seen thought that his/her diagnosis was the right one. Dr. Sherry told Elizabeth that her form of RND, intermittent RND, has the highest success rate for a complete cure. He told her that he would put her on the waiting list for his outpatient treatment program, but that he thought she could cure herself by doing one hour of aerobic exercise everyday.

When Elizabeth and I got home, we remained guarded in our optimism. We both were scared to get our hopes up yet once again, but at the same time she was determined to give this new plan 100% of her effort. She stopped all of her medications except the antidepressant and started her workout program. After three weeks, I called Dr. Sherry to give him an update. I relayed to his nurse that we were not seeing any improvement and that Elizabeth had become very depressed. The day before she had completely "shut down" and refused to eat or speak. Dr. Sherry personally called me back and said that Elizabeth could come to CHOP to start the RND program the very next day. I told him that I would have to let Elizabeth make that decision, as she would have to miss most of her senior end of the year activities. When I told Elizabeth, she looked at me as if I had lost my mind. Of course she wanted to go right away and she would sacrifice missing most of her graduation events. We had just three weeks before her graduation, so we packed our bags and flew to Philadelphia.

Elizabeth can tell you exactly what she went through during her three weeks of treatment at CHOP. I dropped her off at the day hospital every morning and went back to get her in the afternoon, but I do not know firsthand all that her treatment entailed. Dr. Sherry told her on the first day that he was the only person who was allowed to ask her about her pain and the only person she was allowed to tell. She never complained to me and I did my very best not to question her. We planned activities to help take her mind off the pain during treatment, as her pain got worse before it got better.

While I can't tell you exactly what happened during those twelve days of treatment, I can tell you that it worked. Elizabeth got her life back and we got our old Elizabeth back.

We are so grateful to Dr. Sherry and the RND team at CHOP. While Elizabeth and I would like nothing more than to put this all behind us and move forward, we both feel compelled to get the word out and let others know about RND. If we can spare one family from suffering for as long as we did, we will feel like we have made a difference. We have notified every doctor that has treated Elizabeth to let them know the final diagnosis, just in case they ever see another patient with an undiagnosed chronic pain syndrome.

# 11

# *A Sibling's Perspective on RND*

*by Martha Elster*

*I want to be able to take away your pain*
*Even if it means having to endure it myself.*
*I want to be able to fix all of the problems*
*And the obstacles that stand in your way.*
*I want to find a cure for your ailments*
*And help you out in every way.*
*I hate seeing you suffer from pain*
*It kills me to hear you cry and hurt.*
*I know you think the day will never come*
*I wish I could bring it to you sooner*
*But until then please stay strong.*
*I am here to hold you up no matter what.*

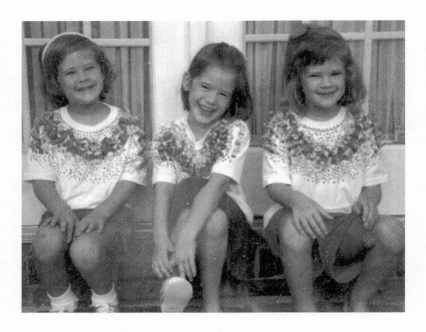

Patricia, Elizabeth, and Martha

Human nature creates a longing within each of us to fix one another's problems and pain. Even seeing a loved one go through the "ouch" caused by something as simple as a skinned knee activates the friend or relative's innate desire to take away each and every possible cause of discomfort. Relief is found in the knowledge that the skinned knee is temporary and is soon soothed by a band-aid. You then create a universal "band-aid" of your love, kindness, and compassion in an attempt to heal every wound. However, what do you do when you realize that this bandage does not conceal *every* relentless and abiding pain?

I certainly never imagined that my reliable "band-aid" would seem an insignificant possibility to my sister as she fought against her impenetrable and unrelenting nemesis, RND, for over three years. For most of my life I had mostly surrendered to the uncontrollable nature of pain, choosing to be more of the introverted observer providing occasional emotional "first aid" when needed. But, suddenly at the age of fourteen I desperately felt the need to become my sister's support and way out of the cycle of pain.

Nevertheless, I found myself faced with a brick wall. Despite my obstinate efforts, I could not become the impossible superhero I so desperately wanted to be for Elizabeth.

However, it would be false to say that my efforts of compassion and love were utterly useless. While I could not provide the golden key to Elizabeth's problems or even find a medicine that would stem the pain, I could give her my unwavering determination and support throughout her struggle.

Since I was unable to create one giant band-aid to encompass all of my sister's problems caused by RND, I began to take small steps and use small band-aids to help her throughout her overall struggle. As a family member or friend of someone suffering from chronic pain, you must realize that the answer to this endless pain cannot be found wholly within you. However, you will become the underlying foundation of strength for your loved one, providing continual love, care, and support in all times of hope and desperation.

So, what do you do?

# The Do's:

1. **Love**.
   Chronic pain can destroy the emotional state of the sufferer and his or her surrounding family. However, love is magic in its hidden powers to heal and mend. Love activates the emotions and feelings necessary to meet the challenges that stand in one's path. Love, overall, restores inner strength within the sufferer to carry on his or her fight.

2. **Support.**
   At times you will feel like there will never be an answer to your loved one's pain. You will wish for a magic wand to resolve the problems instantly. However, your prayers may take time to be answered; so until then, *you* must become the beacon of hope and light for the sufferer. You must provide your relative with enough hope to continue his or her fight against each hurdle.

3. **Simplify.**
   The first thing my sister learned on her road to recovery was that she could not be defeated by her pain. Pain cannot become so unmanageable emotionally that the everyday life and function of an individual is destroyed. You will find that your life changes because of your relative's pain, whether this change is in routine, relationships, or emotional connections. However, you too must not resign your daily life to pain. The key to breaking the cycle of pain, which is fed by time consumption, is to simplify your life in a way that the pain is not able to become a time issue. The most important thing for you to remember is: *Pain is a part of your life and your friend's life, but it is not your whole life.*

4. **Continue.**
   If you do not feel completely committed to supporting your loved one through her uncontrollable tribulations, you need to ask yourself if you are being fair to yourself or your family member. After watching my sister struggle through disintegrating friendships ruptured by her extended hospital stays in other states, I know that the important

thing for her and other chronic pain sufferers is reliability and constant support, not the intermittent care her friends were providing. While the pain should not destroy your own life, you should make yourself at least emotionally available for your friend.

5. **Speak.**

Pain should never be a quiet battle. Thousands suffer from chronic pain syndromes like Elizabeth on a daily basis. Which means you are not alone either; there are dozens of families like yours that experience the same hopes, experiences, and even disappointments. Try to reach out to other sufferers and families in as many ways as possible, such as with the Internet and support groups. Also, it is important to share your struggle with non-pain sufferers in order to increase your community's responsiveness and flexibility towards your loved one. I found the adaptability of Elizabeth's teachers, coaches, and other members of our city a valuable key in helping her both simplify her life and manage her time while in and out of doctors' offices.

6. **Assist.**

Your friend or relative will go to doctor upon doctor, searching for that "golden key" to his or her pain. Do not be afraid to help your friend with his or her quest. While you cannot administer the final answer, you can provide your loved one with the resources she needs to continue her quest for a pain-free life.

# The Don'ts:

1. **Focus.**

   As I said before, ***pain is a part of your life but it is not your whole life***. There will be setbacks in your journey; however, do not focus on the minor pitfalls along the way. You must instead maintain the overall driving force of hope for that ultimate goal of a cure. When your relative or friend loses that focus, you must step in and remind him/her of the final destination. I found that with Elizabeth, frequently saying something as simple as "Go Bee!" (her nickname) was a nonspecific way of reminding her she was not alone while encouraging her to continue her battle.

2. **Blame.**

   It is too easy to point fingers in blame when times get difficult. However, you must remember that chronic pain is not anyone's fault. Humans have absolutely no control over this metamorphic enemy or the power over their lives it will demand as a festering cycle. However, as a friend or family member, you must understand beforehand the emotional and physical needs you will have to meet for your friend.

3. **Discourage.**

   While comments such as "suck it up" and "deal with it" may seem rational ideas initially, they are often hurtful and very discouraging to a chronic pain sufferer. You may have the desire to remind your friend that he or she might have to live with pain forever, but trust me, that is already one of his/her continual fears. I know this is a clichéd saying but stick to it: "If you don't have anything nice to say, don't say anything at all". If you are not going to be a positive influence on your family member or friend, then I advise reconsidering your own feelings towards his/her recovery. It is okay to have discussions with your friend about scenarios such as adapting to lifelong pain in order to calm her fears. However do not focus on these topics negatively or on a regular basis.

4. **Stress.**

Anyone dealing with everyday pain can tell you that it causes a lot of additional stress. Not only does the person have to worry about functioning with the pain, he or she will also be concerned with the looming possibility of not finding an answer or living in pain forever. While you should be primarily concerned with maintaining a "normal" day to day life for the sufferer, you should also try to circumvent any additional unnecessary stressors that may occur. Elizabeth had to learn how to reevaluate her friendships and reduce time spent with friends who constantly emitted drama and tension. As a family, we had to figure out ways to make our home life as stress-free as possible, avoiding unnecessary anxieties such as complaints and meaningless squabbles.

In whatever ways you create "band-aids" to support your loved one, I hope that you are successful. Remember to never lose hope, to "keep going" and "never give up" as you will find yourself urging your friend to do so too. By staying strong through all of the obstacles and disappointments, you will become a role model for your loved one to follow your steps and continue fighting his or her personal battle.

# 12

## *Conclusion: Pain is Relative*

All pain is relative. I'm sure you have heard of the scales for rating pain. I can't count how many times I have been asked to rate my pain. "On a scale of 0-10 what would you rate your pain right now? 0 being no pain, 10 being the worst pain you could possibly imagine." When I first was asked that question I had no idea what to answer. After hearing it dozens of times and really thinking about it, it's a really good system. The doctors and nurses don't take the number you give them and go look it up where a 1 = something, 2 = something, and so forth. They take the number you give them and can say "Wow, her pain is bad. She said that she is feeling a 9 today. That means that her pain must be unbearable today." It gives the health professionals a sense of how you are able to tolerate and function with the amount of pain you are experiencing. It was difficult for me because my pain was intermittent and while I may have had a pain level of 8 or 9 earlier in the day, by the time I saw the doctor my pain could have gone down to a 2 or even 0, no pain. It was also difficult for me to use this scale because I had a tendency to underestimate my pain levels. This is part of having RND, as most RND patients will keep smiling even through pain levels of 8 to 10. So the doctors know that all of pain is relative too, and this scale is the closest they can come to understanding what you feel. There are several different pain scales that are used to quantify a patient's pain level. While I was asked to use a numerical scale from 1-10, younger children are given a visual chart, the Wong-Baker FACES scale, to rate their pain level. There are more complex scales, such as the McGill Pain Index, which takes into account a variety of factors and while it may be more accurate, it takes much longer to administer. The "Pain Scale" sys-

71

tem makes sense in accordance to the last few points I wish to leave you with.

## Point 1: No one else can feel your pain.

It has always bothered me when people who have no idea what I go through on a daily basis say, "I understand." Of course, they don't really understand. They cannot possibly comprehend how intense it is, how it moves all over, how it simply frightens, exhausts, and maddens me. These people, rather, are *trying* to understand. And the ones who really care about you, the people closest to you at heart, they *want* to understand. No one wants to suffer through pain alone. And so, we should give credit to those who are *trying* and *wanting* to understand. That's the closest anyone can get.

Even I can't understand the pain that you go through. Maybe we both have the same diagnosis. That doesn't mean our experiences are the same. Your pain is still unlike mine. I can come closer to understanding, but I can't 100 percent know what you are going through. One girl in the RND program at CHOP described her pain to me as a trapped, hammering pain. But I would describe my pain as stabbing pain. We both had been diagnosed with RND, but it doesn't mean my pain was exactly like hers.

## Point 2: We all feel pain differently.

We all have different experiences with pain. And yes, that is one of the hardest things about diagnosing and treating pain. It is also one of the most frustrating. The worst pain that I have ever felt and can possibly imagine is my chronic pain at its worst. The worst pain that someone else may have ever felt is a broken bone.

But remember Buddha and his First Noble Truth: we will all experience suffering. Mine may not be like yours. For example, you may have RND and your friend may feel no more than a broken bone. Don't compare though. Know that each person you meet or pass by on the street has or will experience some kind of pain. For the person whose worse pain experience was a broken bone that will be their frame of reference for the worst pain they can imagine. It is not until they have a more painful experience, like RND or childbirth, that they will have to re-evaluate their "worst pain". The McGill Pain Index, developed at McGill University by Melzack and Torgerson in 1971, is the closest measure of common human experiences which are the least to most painful.

## Point 3: We all respond to pain differently.

While pain is a universal human experience, each person's response to pain is unique. This is the emotional aspect of chronic pain. The feelings associated with chronic pain cover a wide spectrum from guilt, embarrassment, depression, anger, scared, to outright denial that the pain even exists. Some people are very open and communicative with their feelings about their pain, while others, like me, tend to hide their feelings behind a smile. I could smile through pain at level 9 or 10, just to keep others from worrying about me.

I hope that my story has helped you in some way. Many of us have had to deal with pain for too long. The label of "chronic" demonstrates that. But if currently nothing can be done, no treatments to alleviate the pain, no medicines that work, use this as a time to grow mentally and spiritually. Use this as a time to accept and understand suffering. And if you find that you can learn something, anything, from this experience, you will find that your suffering wasn't in vain.

# 13

## *Journaling*

○ ○ ○ ○ ○ ○ ○ ○ ○ ○ ○ ○ ○ ○ ○ ○ ○ ○ ○ ○ ○ ○ ○ ○ ○ ○ ○ ○ ○ ○ ○ ○ ○

*Confessional writing has been around at least since the Renaissance, but new research suggests that it is far more therapeutic than anyone ever knew ... Researchers found direct physiological evidence [that writing about your feelings and experiences is good for your physical health]: writing increased the level of disease-fighting lymphocytes circulating in the bloodstream. Newsweek, April, 1999*

Researchers, such as James Pennebaker at the University of Texas at Austin, suggest that there are health benefits from journaling. The theory is that regular journaling boosts your immune system. As a result, you are better able to respond to stressful situations without harming your health in any way. So, for chronic pain sufferers, journaling is yet another way to help reduce stress and therefore reduce pain. Journaling can be done by pen and paper, or there is journaling software available for those who prefer to write on the computer.

I strongly encourage you to write down your thoughts and feelings about your pain. You will feel better emotionally and physically when your use journaling as part of your treatment. You will have a written record so that you can see how far you have progressed. Journaling helps you organize your thoughts and focus more clearly on your feelings. You will feel more in control of your feelings when you record them on a regular basis. Journaling will help reduce stress, anxiety, and depression, and the benefit of that will be a reduction in pain. I have some written exercises that you may wish to try to get you started. Remember, your journal is for your eyes only, so keep it in a safe place and feel free to write not only about your feelings about your pain, but also your hopes, dreams, and thoughts about life. Try to keep it upbeat and positive, not dwelling too much on the past, while keeping hope for your future.

For chronic pain sufferers:

1. *How do you feel emotionally? Try to identify a few key words.*

_____

_____

_____

_____

You may feel: scared, alone, depressed, angry. This is all expected. Trust me, whatever word you put down, I've probably been there, along with every other chronic pain sufferer!

2. *How might you change how you feel? What are some activities you can do?*

_____

_____

_____

_____

Hopefully you listed some things that are relaxing for you. Maybe that is taking a bubble bath. Maybe it is reading a book. But don't forget to stay active. With RND staying active is critical. Go out with friends. Go to school every day. It might hurt, but *don't let pain control your life!*

3. *Ask yourself: Do I control my life, or does my pain? What did you do today? Did you keep yourself from doing what you wanted to because you were afraid of the pain?*

_____

_____

_____

_____

I don't blame you if you answered that your pain controls your life. It only makes sense to want to protect yourself from hurting. But do what you can. Don't live in fear. It'll only make you worse.

*4. Does my pain control others around me? Do the people in your life walk on eggshells around you so that they may ease your pain? Does your pain often come up in conversation?*

_____

_____

_____

_____

If you answered "yes," pain is controlling your life. It shouldn't though. Try to live your life as normally as possible. Don't focus on the pain. No one needs to ask you constantly how you feel. If they do, the pain will only become more real.

*5. Are there any specific "triggers" for your pain? Do you find that the same situations are creating stress and increasing your pain? What can you do to change these circumstances?*

_____

_____

_____

_____

As you begin to keep a journal, you will see patterns of situations that increase your pain. These are your "triggers" and once you are aware of them, you can do something to change them.

Any other thoughts you may have you may record below. I also strongly encourage you to keep a journal and write in it daily.

_____

_____

_____

_____

Another method of stress relief you may investigate is seeing someone such as a psychologist to talk to regularly. I saw a doctor mind/body specialist doctor. We met every three weeks and talked about how to try to live healthier and therefore reduce the pain. It was a good way for me to also become more in tune to my body and its needs. Regularly writing in my journal helped me remember things I wanted to talk about when I went to see my doctor. Talking to a professional regularly can help because he or she may be able to see certain stressors or habits that may intensify your pain. These are things that you as the pain sufferer can't always see. So really, don't be afraid to look into seeing someone to talk to on a regular basis.

For those who know someone in pain:

1. *How do you feel when you see your loved one in pain?*

_____

_____

_____

_____

Knowing how you feel will help you understand how you are reacting to your loved one's pain. When you become aware of your own feelings and actions, you can make changes which will help the pain sufferer.

2. *How do you act around the person in pain? Do you act any differently than around others?*

_____

_____

_____

_____

If you act any differently, stop right away! Sometimes (subconsciously) pain patients may find an increase in pain so that they may receive support and pity. I know that you may wish to pamper them and to feel sorry for them, but what we need as pain sufferers is as normal a life as possible.

3. *Do you get annoyed easily from the pain patient's cries and complaints of pain?*

_____

_____

_____

_____

We know you might. We're sorry. But remember that we can't help being in so much pain. And it is impossible to keep it all inside.

4. *What can you do to help keep from getting annoyed?*

_____

_____

_____

_____

This one's up to you. However you choose to "keep your cool", just please, do keep your cool. A ticked off person is the last thing someone who hurts needs to handle.

# 14

## *Keeping a Pain Diary*

Even though it is important to not focus on your illness, you still need to keep a diary of your pain so that you can see patterns and cycles. It also helps when you go to the doctor to have your diary handy, because it is hard to remember accurately your pain cycles and levels from day to day. You will also see if you have progressed from week to week or if one treatment plan is working better than another.

An additional benefit of keeping a pain diary is that you will begin to see that there are times of day when you feel better and have less pain than other times of day. For most people, pain levels tend to be higher later in the day. It is important to note when your best time of day is so that you can schedule important events during those times. You would want to take exams in the morning if that is when you are most pain free, or schedule an interview in the early afternoon if you feel your best after lunch. On the other hand, you might want to schedule a therapy session or a massage in the late afternoon or evening, when you know your pain levels will be higher.

In addition, you might also want to keep a record of medications you take for the pain and how well it works and how long it works. If your pain varies in intensity and/or quality, note descriptive words. If your pain varies in location, note where the pain was each time. Because your pain is chronic, you will be glad if you write these things down, as it is hard to remember what you have tried, what works, and what doesn't. On the next page is a sample chart for documenting your pain.

|  | Pain level and location | How long it lasted | What made it worse | What made it better |
|---|---|---|---|---|
| *Monday* am |  |  |  |  |
| afternoon |  |  |  |  |
| evening |  |  |  |  |
| *Tuesday* am |  |  |  |  |
| afternoon |  |  |  |  |
| evening |  |  |  |  |
| *Wednesday* am |  |  |  |  |
| afternoon |  |  |  |  |
| evening |  |  |  |  |
| *Thursday* am |  |  |  |  |
| afternoon |  |  |  |  |
| evening |  |  |  |  |
| *Friday* am |  |  |  |  |
| afternoon |  |  |  |  |
| evening |  |  |  |  |
| *Saturday* am |  |  |  |  |
| afternoon |  |  |  |  |
| evening |  |  |  |  |
| *Sunday* am |  |  |  |  |
| afternoon |  |  |  |  |
| evening |  |  |  |  |

# RND Resources

For more a general overview of RND by Dr. David Sherry,
**http://www.childhoodrnd.org/media/AMP_RNDparentHandout.pdf**

A video on Reflex Neurovascular Dystrophy in children is available through the Childhood RND Educational Foundation,
**http://www.childhoodrnd.org**.

For more information, contact the Reflex Sympathetic Dystrophy Syndrome Association, at 877-662-7737 or visit **http://www.rsds.org**

A support group for parents of teens with RND which can be found at:
**http://.groups.google.com/group/rsdteenparents**

Information about RND treatment centers:
Children's Hospital of Philadelphia:

| | |
|---|---|
| Address: | 34th Street and Civic Center Boulevard |
| | Philadelphia, PA 19104 |
| Telephone: | 215-590-1000 |
| Website: | **http://www.chop.edu** |

Seattle Children's Hospital:

| | |
|---|---|
| Address: | 4800 Sand Point Way NE |
| | Seattle, WA 98105 |
| Telephone: | 206-987-2000 |
| Website: | **http://www.seattlechildrens.org** |

## The Children's Institute of Pittsburgh:

| | |
|---|---|
| Address: | 1405 Shady Avenue |
| | Pittsburgh, PE 15217-1350 |
| Telephone: | 412-420-2400 |
| Website: | **http://www.amazingkids.org/dg_16.asp** |

## Frazier Rehab Institute:

| | |
|---|---|
| Address: | 220 Abraham Flexner Way |
| | Louisville, KY 40202 |
| Telephone: | 502-582-7400 |
| Website: | **http://www.jewishhospital.org/healthnetwork/frazier** |

## Legacy Emanuel Children's Hospital

| | |
|---|---|
| Address: | 2801 N Gantenbein Avenue |
| | Portland, OR 97227 |
| Telephone: | 503-413-2200 |
| Website: | **http://www.legacyhealth.org/homepage.cfm** |

# Triplets Who Care, Inc.

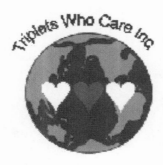

Triplets Who Care, Inc. is a not-for-profit organization started by my sisters and me. Through Triplets Who Care, Inc. we create awareness about causes of our choice and help give aid in some form. To learn more visit our website:

www.TripletsWhoCare.org

Order a "Power Through Pain" wristband! I wear mine every day, and it reminds me that there are others out there who suffer from chronic pain and that I can help them. By ordering a bracelet you can help too. The money raised from the bracelets will be donated to RND research and education. There is an order form at the end of this book or use these links to order online:

www.TripletsWhoCare.org/RND

www.TripletsWhoCare.org/Power_Through_Pain

# *About The Author*

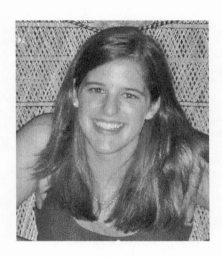

Elizabeth Elster is a college student at Washington University in St. Louis. She was born and raised in Winston-Salem, NC along with her triplet sisters and older brother. Her father is a radiologist and her mother is a teacher. Despite having access to a wealth of information and health care, it took three and a half years for Elizabeth's mysterious pain to be identified and treated. It was during her high school years that she suffered from a chronic pain condition known as Reflex Neurovascular Dystrophy, or RND. While suffering from her own pain, however, Elizabeth was able to focus her time and attention to helping others. She volunteered over 500 hours of her time to the community and received the Congressional Gold Medal for her efforts. In addition to academics and volunteer work, Elizabeth was a member of the varsity swim team, serving as captain her senior year. Elizabeth has continued these interests in college. She is a member of the women's water polo team and a member of the Alpha Phi Omega service fraternity.

This book chronicles Elizabeth's journey through high school trying to find a cause and a cure for her then unknown pain disorder. This experience changed Elizabeth's life and her long term goals. She is studying pre-med and plans to become a pediatric rheumatologist. Her ambition is to one day treat others with RND.

# References

Amplified Musculoskeletal Pain in Childhood. Diagnosis and Treatment. A Guide for Physical and Occupational Therapists. (Videotape, DVD) MMII, Sherry DD, executive producer. www.childhoodrnd.org

Bernstein BH, Singsen BH, Kent JT, Kornreich H, King K, Hicks R, Hanson V. Reflex neurovascular dystrophy in childhood. *Journal of Pedatrics* 1978;93:211-215.

Cohen AM, Kemp S, Perkins TER. The physiotherapy management of reflex sympathetic dystrophy. Arch Dis Child 2000;82(Suppl. 1):A45.

Murray CS, Cohen A, Perkins T, Davidson JE, Sills JA. Morbidity in reflex sympathetic dystrophy. Arch Dis Child 2000;82:231-3.

Sherry DD. An overview of amplified musculoskeletal pain syndromes *J Rheumatol* 2000;Suppl 58:44-48.

Sherry D, Malleson PN. The idiopathic musculoskeletal pain syndromes in childhood. Rheum Dis North Am. 2002 Aug;28(3):669-85.

Sherry DD, McGuire T, Salmonson K, Wallace CA, Mellins E, Nepom B. Psychosomatic musculoskeletal pain in childhood: clinical and psychological analysis of one hundred children. *Pediatrics* 1991;88:1093-1099.

Sherry, DD. Pain Syndromes. In: Isenberg DA, Miller JJ III (eds). Adolescent Rheumatology, London, Martin Duntz LTD. 1998, p 197-227.

Sherry DD, Wallace CA, Kelley C, Kidder M, Sapp L. Short and long term outcome of children with complex regional pain syndrome type I treated with exercise therapy. *Clin J Pain* 1999;15:218-223.

Sherry DD, Weisman R. Psychological aspects of childhood reflex neurovascular dystrophy. *Pediatrics* 1988;81:572-578.

# *Wristband Order Form*
# *Power Through Pain*

*Wristband
Order Form*

*$2.00 each*

Name: _____

Address: _____

City, State, Zip: _____

Quantity _____ @ $2 each                    $_____

Shipping and Handling                               $ 3.00

Total                                                        $_____

Mail Check or Money Order made payable to Triplets Who Care, Inc to:

Triplets Who Care, Inc
3131 Milhaven Lake Dr
Winston-Salem, NC 27106

# *Book Order Form*
# *Power Through Pain*

*Order Form*

Name: _____

Address: _____

City, State, Zip: _____

Quantity: _____ @ $12.95 each          $_____

Shipping and Handling                          $_____

       1-5 copies     $5.95

       6-10 copies    9.95

       11-20 copies  14.95

       21 or more   19.95

Total                                                    $_____

Make check payable to Triplets Who Care, Inc and mail to:

      Triplets Who Care, Inc
      3131 Milhaven Lake Dr
      Winston-Salem, NC 27106

978-0-595-43716-0
0-595-43716-8

Made in the USA
Lexington, KY
12 April 2014